DASH DIET COOKBOOK

BOOKS BY THE AUTHOR
The Complete Mediterranean Diet Cookbook For Beginners
The Complete Plant-Based Diet Cookbook
The Anti-inflammatory Diet Kitchen Cookbook For Beginners
Intermittent Fasting For Women Over
Keto Crockpot Recipes Cookbook
The Complete Slow Cooker Cookbook
The Super Easy Heart-healthy Cookbook

DASH DIET COOKBOOK

Healthy Delicious Recipes to Lower Blood Pressure,Boost Metabolism and Improve Your Health

By

Sabestian Gastronomer

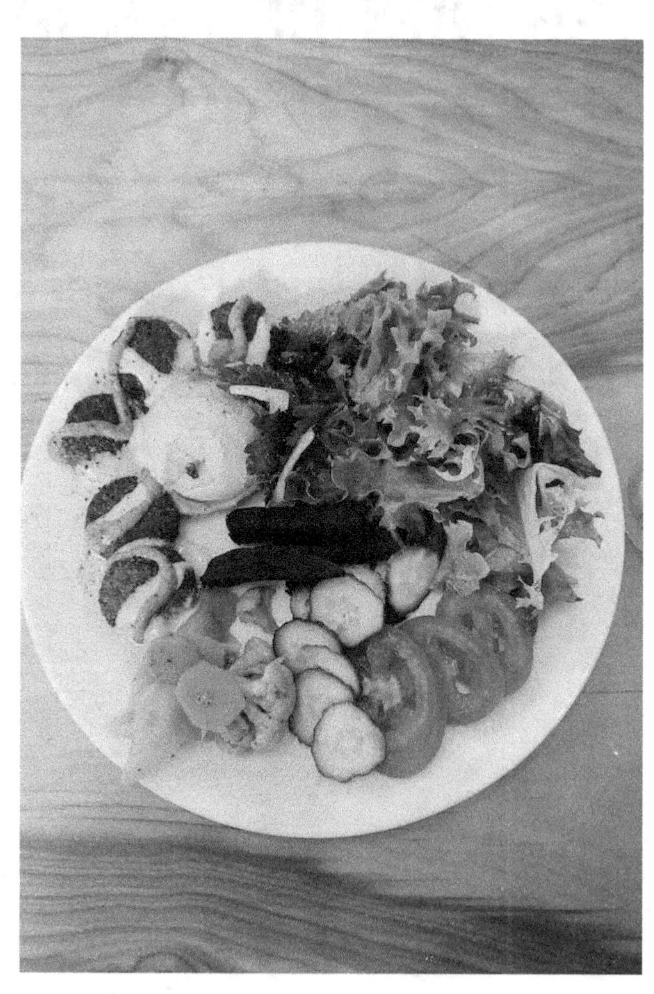

TABLE OF CONTENT

"Fuel your body with the vibrant colors of the DASH diet, and watch your health soar. Every bite is a step towards a stronger, happier you."

"Embrace the power of DASH - Discipline, Action, and Sustained Health. Let each nutritious choice be a testament to your commitment to a life well-lived."

FORWARD

The DASH (Dietary Approaches to Stop Hypertension) diet has gained widespread recognition for its effectiveness in promoting heart health and managing hypertension. Developed by the National Heart, Lung, and Blood Institute (NHLBI), the DASH diet emphasizes a balanced and nutrient-rich approach to eating, with a particular focus on reducing sodium intake.

Numerous individuals have reported significant benefits from adopting the DASH diet. One of the key aspects contributing to its popularity is its proven ability to lower blood pressure. By encouraging the consumption of fruits, vegetables, whole grains, lean proteins, and low-fat dairy, while minimizing the intake of saturated fats and sodium, the DASH diet promotes overall cardiovascular well-being.

Many people have found success in managing their blood pressure and overall health by following the principles outlined in the DASH diet. Research studies have consistently shown that adherence to the DASH eating plan can contribute to lower blood pressure levels, making it an invaluable resource for individuals with hypertension or those aiming to prevent its onset.

Personally, the DASH diet has been beneficial for me as well. Adopting a lifestyle that aligns with the DASH principles has not only improved my blood pressure but has also led to an overall sense of well-being. The emphasis on whole, nutrient-dense foods has positively impacted my energy levels, weight management, and cardiovascular health. It's not just a temporary fix but rather a sustainable approach to eating that promotes long-term health benefits.

In addition to its impact on blood pressure, the DASH diet is often praised for its flexibility and accessibility. It doesn't require special foods or complicated meal plans, making it practical for a wide range of individuals. The emphasis on a variety of food groups ensures that followers can enjoy a diverse and satisfying diet while reaping the health rewards associated with this evidence-based approach.

The DASH diet has proven to be a valuable resource for many, offering a realistic and effective way to manage hypertension and promote heart health. Its widespread success is attributed to its simplicity, emphasis on whole foods, and scientifically supported impact on blood pressure levels. As with any dietary approach, individual experiences may vary, but the overall positive outcomes reported by many highlight the significance of the DASH diet in the realm of cardiovascular health.

INTRODUCTION

Welcome to the flavorful journey towards a healthier and heart-conscious lifestyle with our DASH Diet Cookbook. This culinary guide is designed to be your trusted companion on the path to better well-being, offering a delectable array of recipes that align with the principles of the Dietary Approaches to Stop Hypertension (DASH) diet. In these pages, you'll discover a treasure trove of dishes crafted with the perfect blend of taste and nutrition, making it easier than ever to embrace a heart-healthy way of eating.

Inside this cookbook, you'll find a diverse collection of recipes ranging from breakfast delights to satisfying dinners, all thoughtfully curated to support your journey toward optimal cardiovascular health. The DASH diet emphasizes the consumption of nutrient-rich foods, such as fruits, vegetables, lean proteins, whole grains, and low-fat dairy, while minimizing sodium intake and steering clear of excessive saturated fats.

But this cookbook is more than just a collection of recipes – it's a comprehensive guide to understanding and implementing the DASH diet in your daily life. We provide practical tips, substitution suggestions, and meal planning advice to help you seamlessly incorporate these heart-healthy principles into your routine. Whether you're a seasoned home chef or just starting your culinary adventures, our cookbook is crafted to suit all skill levels, ensuring that everyone can enjoy the benefits of the DASH diet.

As the creator of this cookbook, I can personally attest to the transformative power of the DASH diet. The journey toward adopting this approach to eating has not only positively impacted my cardiovascular health but has also enhanced my overall well-being. Through the delicious recipes within these pages, I aim to share the joy of nutritious and flavorful meals that have played a pivotal role in my own health journey.

But the success of the DASH diet extends beyond my personal experience. Countless individuals have embraced this dietary approach and witnessed significant improvements in their blood pressure, weight management, and overall health. The testimonials and success stories from those who have incorporated the DASH diet into their lives serve as a testament to its efficacy and long-lasting impact.

So, embark on this culinary adventure with us, savoring the delightful flavors of health and vitality. Let this cookbook be your guide to a heart-conscious lifestyle, where every meal brings you one step closer to a healthier and happier you.

Tips for Successful DASH Diet Cooking

The DASH (Dietary Approaches to Stop Hypertension) diet is known for promoting heart health by emphasizing nutrient-rich foods and controlling sodium intake. Here are some tips for successful DASH diet cooking:

Prioritize Fresh Produce:

Base your meals on a variety of fruits and vegetables. Aim for colorful options to ensure a diverse range of vitamins, minerals, and antioxidants.

Choose Lean Proteins:

Lean protein options include fish, chicken, beans, and lentils. They support a balanced diet and are vital for the health of muscles.

Include Whole Grains:

Choose whole grains over refined grains, such as quinoa, brown rice, and whole wheat bread. Fiber from whole grains promotes healthy digestion and blood sugar regulation.

Limit Sodium Intake:

Be mindful of sodium content in your ingredients. Use herbs, spices, and other seasonings to add flavor instead of relying on excessive salt. This is crucial for managing blood pressure.

Healthy Fats:

Incorporate foods like avocados, almonds, seeds, and olive oil that are good sources of fat. When these fats are eaten in moderation, they are good for heart health.

Watch Portion Sizes:

Be aware of portion control to avoid overeating. Use smaller plates and bowls to help regulate the amount of food you consume while still feeling satisfied.

Cook at Home:

Prepare meals at home whenever possible. This allows you to have better control over the ingredients and cooking methods, reducing the likelihood of hidden sodium and unhealthy fats.

Experiment with Herbs and Spices:

Enhance the flavor of your dishes with a variety of herbs and spices. This not only adds taste but also provides additional health benefits.

Stay Hydrated:

Water is essential for overall health. Drink plenty of water throughout the day, and consider incorporating water-rich foods like fruits and vegetables into your meals.

Plan Ahead:

Plan your meals and snacks in advance to ensure a well-balanced and DASH-friendly diet. This can also help you resist the temptation of unhealthy, convenience foods.

Moderate Alcohol Consumption:

If you do drink, make sure to do it in moderation. This usually translates to a maximum of one drink for women and a maximum of two for men per day.

Be Mindful of Added Sugars:

Eat fewer foods and drinks that have a lot of added sugar. To sate your sweet taste, go for naturally sweet fruits or natural sweeteners like honey.

By incorporating these tips into your cooking routine, you can create delicious and heart-healthy meals that align with the principles of the DASH diet.

Recommended Servings and Portions

The serving sizes are based on a standard 2,000-calorie per day diet. Adjustments may be necessary based on factors such as age, gender, and activity level.

Here are the recommended servings for key food groups in the DASH diet:

Grains:

- 6-8 servings per day
- Examples of one serving: 1 slice of whole wheat bread, 1/2 cup of cooked brown rice or quinoa.

Vegetables:

- 4-5 servings per day

- Examples of one serving: 1 cup of raw leafy greens, 1/2 cup of cooked vegetables.

Fruits:
  - 4-5 servings per day
  - Examples of one serving: 1 medium-sized fruit (e.g., apple, banana), 1/2 cup of fresh fruit, or 4 ounces of 100% fruit juice.

Dairy (Low-Fat or Fat-Free):
  - 2-3 servings per day
  - Examples of one serving: 1 cup of low-fat or fat-free milk, 1 cup of yogurt, or 1.5 ounces of cheese.

Lean Protein (Meat, Poultry, Fish, Nuts, Seeds, Legumes):
  - 2 or fewer servings of lean meat, poultry, or fish per day
  - Examples of one serving: 3 ounces of cooked lean meat, poultry, or fish; 1/2 cup of cooked legumes; 1 egg; 1 ounce of nuts or seeds.

Fats and Oils:
  - Two or fewer servings per day
  - Examples of one serving: 1 teaspoon of olive oil, 1 tablespoon of salad dressing, or 1/8 of an avocado.

Sweets:
  - Five or fewer servings per week
  - Examples of one serving: one tablespoon of sugar, 1 tablespoon of jam or jelly, or 1/2 cup of sorbet.

Nuts, Seeds, and Legumes:
  - 4-5 servings per week
   - Examples of one serving: 1/3 cup of nuts, 2 tablespoons of seeds, or 1/2 cup of cooked legumes.

Remember to adjust these recommendations based on individual calorie needs and health goals.

Choosing DASH-Friendly Ingredients

When selecting ingredients for DASH (Dietary Approaches to Stop Hypertension) diet-friendly meals, it's essential to focus on nutrient-dense, whole foods while limiting sodium and saturated fat. Here's a guide to choosing DASH diet-friendly ingredients:

Fruits and Vegetables:
  - Choose a variety of colorful fruits and vegetables.
  - Opt for fresh or frozen options without added sauces or salts.
   - Experiment with leafy greens, berries, citrus fruits, tomatoes, and cruciferous vegetables.

Whole Grains:
   - Select whole grains like brown rice, quinoa, oats, barley, and whole wheat.
  - Check labels to ensure minimal processing and added sugars.

Lean Proteins:

- Include lean sources of protein such as skinless poultry, fish, lean cuts of beef or pork, tofu, beans, and legumes.

- Limit processed meats and choose cooking methods like grilling, baking, or steaming.

Low-Fat or Fat-Free Dairy:

- Choose dairy products that are reduced in fat or fat free, such as yogurt, cheese, and milk.

- Use plain yogurt with fresh fruit on top for natural sweetness.

Healthy Fats:

- Use heart-healthy fats from nuts, seeds, avocados, and olive oil.

- Minimize the amount of trans and saturated fats in processed and fried foods.

Nuts, Seeds, and Legumes:

- Incorporate unsalted nuts and seeds for healthy fats and protein.

- Include legumes such as lentils, chickpeas, and black beans for fiber and protein.

Herbs and Spices:

- Flavor dishes with herbs and spices instead of excessive salt.

- Experiment with garlic, basil, thyme, rosemary, turmeric, and other flavorful options.

Seafood:

- For omega-3 fatty acids, choose for fatty fish like trout, salmon, and mackerel.

- Try to have two or more servings of fish per week.

Whole Food Snacks:

- Snack on whole foods like fresh fruit, vegetables with hummus, or a small handful of nuts.

- Avoid processed snacks high in salt, sugar, and unhealthy fats.

Beverages

- Sip lots of water during the day.

- Minimize sugary drinks and substitute flavorful herbal teas or infused water.

Sodium-Conscious Choices:

- Select low-sodium or no-salt-added canned goods.

- Be mindful of condiments and choose low-sodium versions.

Sweeteners:

- Use natural sweeteners like honey, maple syrup, or agave in moderation.

- Minimize added sugars by focusing on the natural sweetness of fruits.

Portion-Controlled Options:

- Recognize portion sizes to control total caloric consumption.

- Use smaller dishes and plates to assist with portion management.

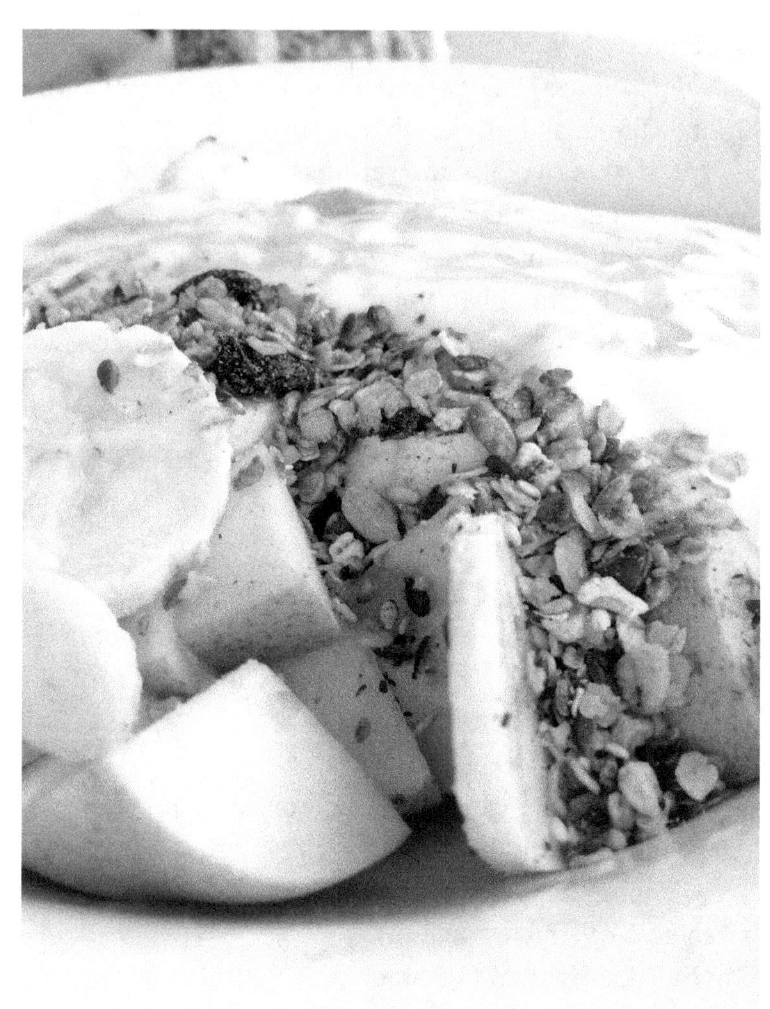

CHAPTER 1: BREAKFAST DELIGHT

Greek Yogurt Parfait

Ingredients:
- 1 cup nonfat Greek yogurt
- 1/2 cup mixed berries (blueberries, strawberries)
- 1 tablespoon honey
- 1/4 cup granola

Preparation:
1. Layer the Greek yogurt, in a bowl or glass
2. Add a layer of mixed berries.
3. Drizzle honey over the berries.
4. Top with granola for crunch.
5. Repeat layers if desired.

Vegetable Omelet

Ingredients:
- 2 eggs
- 1/4 cup diced bell peppers
- 1/4 cup diced tomatoes
- 1/4 cup chopped spinach
- Salt and pepper to taste

Preparation:
1. Whisk eggs in a bowl and season with salt and pepper.

2. In a non-stick pan, sauté vegetables until tender.

3. Pour whisked eggs over vegetables.

4. Cook until the edges set, then flip and cook the other side.

Overnight Chia Pudding

Ingredients:
- 2 tablespoons chia seeds
- 1 cup unsweetened almond milk
- 1/2 teaspoon vanilla extract
- 1 tablespoon maple syrup
- Fresh fruit for topping

Preparation:
1. Mix chia seeds, almond milk, vanilla extract, and maple syrup in a jar.
2. Refrigerate overnight.
3. Top with fresh fruit before serving.

Quinoa Breakfast Bowl

Ingredients:
- 1/2 cup cooked quinoa
- 1/4 cup sliced almonds
- 1/2 cup sliced banana
- 1 tablespoon honey
- A pinch of cinnamon

Preparation:
1. Mix cooked quinoa with sliced almonds.
2. Top with banana slices.
3. Drizzle honey and sprinkle cinnamon.

Avocado Toast

Ingredients:
- 1 slice whole-grain bread
- 1/2 ripe avocado
- Cherry tomatoes, sliced
- Salt and pepper to taste

Preparation:
1. Toast the bread slice.
2. Mash avocado and spread it on the toast.
3. Top with sliced cherry tomatoes.
4. Season with salt and pepper.

Berry Smoothie Bowl

Ingredients:
- One cup of mixed berries like: (strawberries, blueberries, raspberries)
- 1/2 banana
- 1/2 cup low-fat yogurt
- 1 tablespoon chia seeds
- Granola for topping

Preparation:
1. Blend berries, banana, and yogurt until smooth.
2. Pour into a bowl.
3. Top with chia seeds and granola.

Spinach and Feta Breakfast Wrap

Ingredients:
- Whole-grain tortilla
- 2 eggs, scrambled
- Handful of fresh spinach
- 2 tablespoons feta cheese
- Salsa for topping

Preparation:
1. Fill the tortilla with scrambled eggs, spinach, and feta.
2. Roll it up and warm in a pan.
3. Top with salsa.

Cottage Cheese and Fruit Bowl

Ingredients:
- 1/2 cup low-fat cottage cheese
- Pineapple chunks
- Grapes, halved
- Walnuts for crunch

Preparation:
1. Combine cottage cheese with pineapple and grapes.
2. Top with walnuts.

Whole Wheat Pancakes

Ingredients:
- 1 cup whole wheat flour
- 1 tablespoon baking powder
- 1 egg
- 1 cup skim milk
- Berries for topping

Preparation:
1. Mix flour, baking powder, egg, and milk in a bowl.
2. Cook pancakes on a griddle.
3. Top with fresh berries.

Sweet Potato Hash

Ingredients:
- 1 sweet potato, grated
- 1/4 cup diced onion
- 1/4 cup bell peppers
- 1 tablespoon olive oil
- Poached egg for topping

Preparation:
1. Sauté sweet potato, onion, and bell peppers in olive oil until cooked.
2. Top with a poached egg.

Apple Cinnamon Oatmeal

Ingredients:
- 1/2 cup rolled oats
- 1 cup unsweetened almond milk
- 1 apple, diced
- 1/2 teaspoon cinnamon
- Nuts for topping

Preparation:
1. Cook oats with almond milk, diced apple, and cinnamon.
2. Top with nuts.

Smoked Salmon Bagel

Ingredients:
- Whole grain bagel
- 2 oz smoked salmon
- Cream cheese
- Capers and red onion slices

Preparation:
1. Toast the bagel.
2. Spread cream cheese on each half.
3. Top with smoked salmon, capers, and red onion slices.

Enjoy your DASH diet-friendly breakfasts!

CHAPTER 2: SOUPS AND SALADS

Minestrone Soup

Ingredients:
- 1 cup diced carrots
- 1 cup chopped celery
- 1 cup diced zucchini
- 1 cup green beans, chopped
- 1 can (15 oz) kidney beans, drained and rinsed
- 1 can (15 oz) diced tomatoes
- 4 cups low-sodium vegetable broth
- 1 teaspoon dried oregano
- 1 teaspoon dried basil
- Salt and pepper to taste

Preparation:

1. In a large pot, combine all the vegetables, beans, tomatoes, and vegetable broth.

2. Add oregano, basil, salt, and pepper.

3. Bring to a boil, then reduce heat and simmer until vegetables are tender.

4. Adjust seasoning as needed before serving.

Lentil and Vegetable Stew

Ingredients:
- 1 cup dried green lentils
- 1 onion, diced
- 2 carrots, sliced
- 2 celery stalks, chopped
- 3 cloves garlic, minced
- 1 can (14 oz) diced tomatoes
- 4 cups low-sodium vegetable broth
- 1 teaspoon ground cumin
- 1 teaspoon paprika
- Salt and pepper to taste

Preparation:
1. Rinse lentils and combine with all vegetables, tomatoes, and vegetable broth in a pot.
2. Add cumin, paprika, salt, and pepper.
3. Bring to a boil, then simmer until lentils are cooked and vegetables are tender.
4. Adjust seasoning before serving.

Chicken and Vegetable Soup

Ingredients:
- 1 lb boneless, skinless chicken breast, diced
- 1 onion, chopped
- 2 carrots, sliced
- 2 celery stalks, diced
- 1 cup green beans, chopped

- 4 cups low-sodium chicken broth
- 1 teaspoon dried thyme
- 1 teaspoon garlic powder
- Salt and pepper to taste

Preparation:

1. In a large pot, cook chicken until browned. Add onions, carrots, and celery.
2. Add the chicken broth and heat it until it boils.
3. Add green beans, thyme, garlic powder, salt, and pepper.
4. Simmer until vegetables are tender and flavors meld.

Quinoa and Vegetable Stew

Ingredients:
- 1 cup quinoa, rinsed
- 1 onion, diced
- 2 carrots, sliced
- 2 bell peppers, chopped
- 3 cloves garlic, minced
- 4 cups low-sodium vegetable broth
- One can (15 oz) of rinsed and drained chickpeas
- 1 teaspoon cumin
- 1 teaspoon smoked paprika
- Salt and pepper to taste

Preparation:

1. Combine quinoa, vegetables, garlic, and vegetable broth in a pot.

2. Add chickpeas, cumin, paprika, salt, and pepper.

3. Bring to a boil, then simmer until quinoa is cooked and vegetables are tender.

4. Adjust seasoning before serving.

Turkey and Bean Chili

Ingredients:
- 1 lb ground turkey
- 1 onion, chopped
- 2 bell peppers, diced
- Two cans (15 oz each) of washed and drained kidney beans
- 1 can (28 oz) crushed tomatoes
- 2 cups low-sodium chicken broth
- 2 teaspoons chili powder
- 1 teaspoon cumin
- Salt and pepper to taste

Preparation:
1. In a pot, cook ground turkey until browned. Add onions and bell peppers.

2. Stir in kidney beans, crushed tomatoes, chicken broth, chili powder, cumin, salt, and pepper.

3. Simmer until flavors meld and chili thickens.

Spinach and White Bean Soup

Ingredients:
- 1 onion, chopped
- 2 carrots, sliced
- 3 cloves garlic, minced
- One can (15 oz) of washed and drained cannellini beans
- 4 cups low-sodium vegetable broth
- 4 cups fresh spinach leaves
- 1 teaspoon dried thyme
- Salt and pepper to taste

Preparation:
1. Sauté onions, carrots, and garlic until softened in a pot.
2. Add cannellini beans, vegetable broth, spinach, thyme, salt, and pepper.
3. Simmer until spinach wilts and flavors combine.

Butternut Squash Soup

Ingredients:
- 1 butternut squash, peeled and diced
- 1 onion, chopped
- 2 carrots, sliced
- 4 cups low-sodium vegetable broth
- 1 teaspoon ground cinnamon
- 1/2 teaspoon nutmeg
- Salt and pepper to taste

Preparation:

1. In a pot, combine butternut squash, onions, carrots, and vegetable broth.

2. Add cinnamon, nutmeg, salt, and pepper.

3. Simmer until squash is tender, then blend until smooth.

Shrimp and Vegetable Stew

Ingredients:

- 1 lb shrimp, peeled and deveined
- 1 onion, diced
- 2 bell peppers, chopped
- 1 zucchini, sliced
- 1 can (14 oz) diced tomatoes
- 4 cups low-sodium vegetable broth
- 1 teaspoon dried basil
- 1 teaspoon Old Bay seasoning
- Salt and pepper to taste

Preparation:

1. Cook shrimp in a pot until pink. Add onions, bell peppers, and zucchini.

2. Pour in diced tomatoes and vegetable broth.

3. Season with basil, Old Bay, salt, and pepper.

4. Simmer until vegetables are tender.

Cabbage and Tomato Soup

Ingredients:
- 1 small head cabbage, shredded
- 1 onion, chopped
- 2 carrots, sliced
- 1 can (14 oz) crushed tomatoes
- 4 cups low-sodium vegetable broth
- 1 teaspoon dried thyme
- 1 teaspoon paprika
- Salt and pepper to taste

Preparation:
1. Sauté onions, carrots, and cabbage until softened in a pot.
2. Add crushed tomatoes, vegetable broth, thyme, paprika, salt, and pepper.
3. Simmer until the cabbage is tender.

Sweet Potato and Black Bean Soup

Ingredients:
- 2 sweet potatoes, peeled and diced
- 1 onion, chopped
- One can (15 oz) of rinsed and drained black beans
- 4 cups low-sodium vegetable broth
- 1 teaspoon ground cumin
- 1 teaspoon smoked paprika
- Salt and pepper to taste

Preparation:

1. In a pot, combine sweet potatoes, onions, black beans, and vegetable broth.
2. Add cumin, paprika, salt, and pepper.
3. Simmer until sweet potatoes are tender.

Tomato Basil Soup

Ingredients:

- 1 can (28 oz) crushed tomatoes
- 1 onion, chopped
- 3 cloves garlic, minced
- 4 cups low-sodium vegetable broth
- 1 cup fresh basil leaves, chopped
- 1 teaspoon dried oregano
- Salt and pepper to taste

Preparation:

1. Sauté onions and garlic until softened in a pot.
2. Add crushed tomatoes, vegetable broth, basil, oregano, salt, and pepper.
3. Simmer until flavors meld

Barley and Mushroom Stew

Ingredients:

- 1 cup barley, rinsed
- 1 lb mushrooms, sliced
- 1 onion, diced

- 4 cups low-sodium vegetable broth
- 2 teaspoons soy sauce
- 1 teaspoon dried thyme
- Salt and pepper to taste

Preparation:

1. Sauté mushrooms and onions until tender in a pot.

2. Add barley, vegetable broth, soy sauce, thyme, salt, and pepper.

3. Simmer until the barley is cooked and flavors meld.

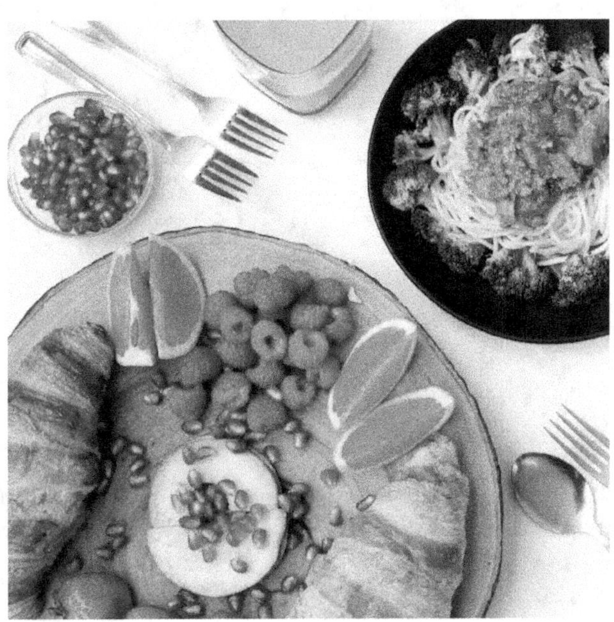

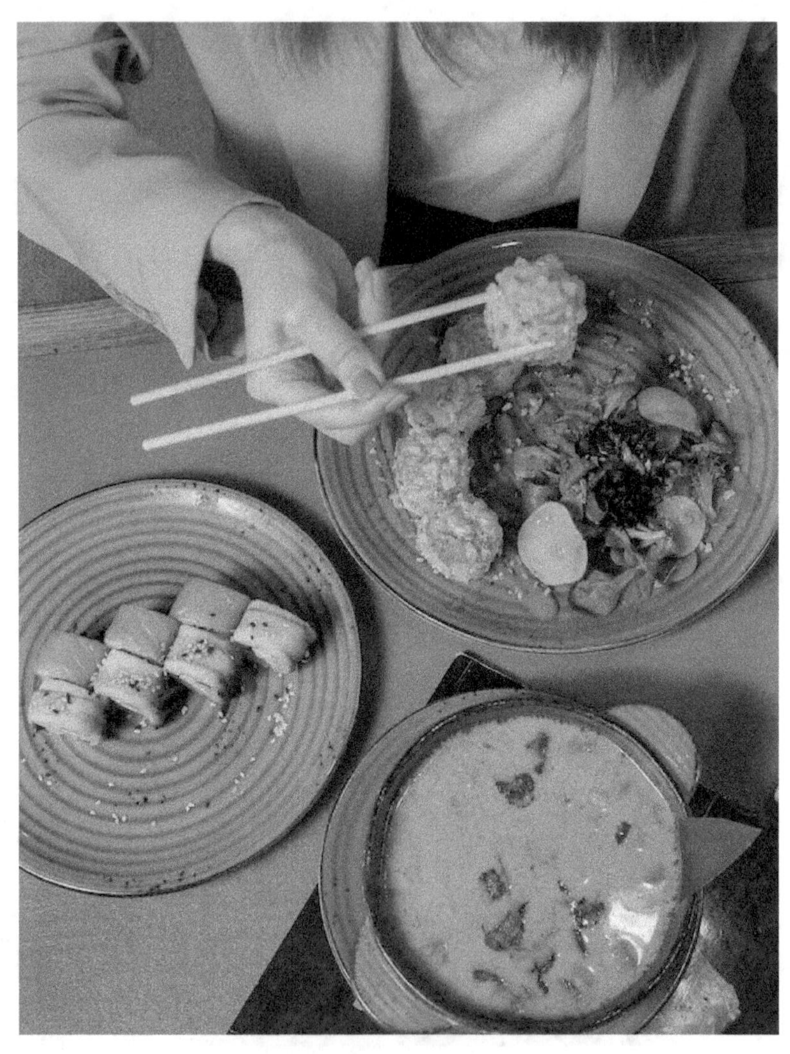

CHAPTER 3: MAIN COURSE

Grilled Lemon Herb Chicken

Ingredients:
- 4 boneless, skinless chicken breasts
- 2 lemons (juiced)
- 2 tablespoons olive oil
- 2 cloves garlic (minced)
- 1 teaspoon dried oregano
- Salt and pepper to taste

Preparation:
1. In a bowl, mix lemon juice, olive oil, minced garlic, oregano, salt, and pepper.
2. Marinate chicken breasts in the mixture for at least 30 minutes.
3. Grill chicken until fully cooked, about 6-8 minutes per side.

Quinoa Salad with Mixed Vegetables

Ingredients:
- 1 cup quinoa (cooked)
- 1 cup cherry tomatoes (halved)
- 1 cucumber (diced)
- 1 bell pepper (diced)

- 1/4 cup red onion (finely chopped)
- 2 tablespoons olive oil
- 2 tablespoons balsamic vinegar
- Salt and pepper to taste

Preparation:

1. In a large bowl, combine cooked quinoa, cherry tomatoes, cucumber, bell pepper, and red onion.
2. Combine the olive oil, balsamic vinegar, salt, and pepper in a small bowl.
3. Toss the salad with the dressing until well combined.

Baked Salmon with Dill

Ingredients:
- 4 salmon filets
- 2 tablespoons fresh dill (chopped)
- 1 lemon (sliced)
- 2 cloves garlic (minced)
- Salt and pepper to taste

Preparation:

1. Preheat the oven to 375°F (190°C).
2. Arrange the filets of salmon on a baking pan.
3. Season with minced garlic, chopped dill, salt, and pepper.
4. Top each filet with lemon slices.
5. Bake for 15-20 minutes or until salmon flakes easily with a fork.

Lentil and Vegetable Soup

Ingredients:
1 cup dry green lentils (rinsed)
1 onion (chopped)
2 carrots (diced)
2 celery stalks (chopped)
3 cloves garlic (minced)
1 can (14 oz) diced tomatoes
6 cups vegetable broth
1 teaspoon cumin
1 teaspoon thyme
Salt and pepper to taste

Preparation:
Add the onions, carrots, celery, and garlic to a large pot and sauté until softened.
Add lentils, diced tomatoes, vegetable broth, cumin, thyme, salt, and pepper.
Simmer for 25-30 minutes or until lentils are tender.

Turkey and Vegetable Skewers

Ingredients:
1 pound lean turkey breast (cut into cubes)
1 zucchini (sliced)
1 bell pepper (sliced)
1 red onion (sliced)
2 tablespoons olive oil
1 teaspoon paprika

1 teaspoon garlic powder

Salt and pepper to taste

Preparation:

Preheat grill or oven broiler.

In a bowl, toss turkey cubes, zucchini, bell pepper, and red onion with olive oil, paprika, garlic powder, salt, and pepper.

Thread onto skewers and grill for 10-15 minutes, turning occasionally.

Spinach and Feta Stuffed Chicken Breast

Ingredients:

4 boneless, skinless chicken breasts

2 cups fresh spinach (chopped)

1/2 cup feta cheese (crumbled)

2 tablespoons olive oil

1 teaspoon dried oregano

Salt and pepper to taste

Preparation:

Preheat the oven to 400°F (200°C).

In a bowl, mix chopped spinach, feta, olive oil, dried oregano, salt, and pepper.

Cut a pocket into each chicken breast and stuff with the spinach and feta mixture.

Bake the chicken for 25 to 30 minutes, or until it is thoroughly done.

Sweet Potato and Black Bean Chili

Ingredients:

2 sweet potatoes (peeled and diced)

One can (15 oz) of rinsed and drained black beans

1 can (14 oz) diced tomatoes

1 onion (chopped)

2 cloves garlic (minced)

2 teaspoons chili powder

1 teaspoon cumin

1/2 teaspoon smoked paprika

Salt and pepper to taste

Preparation:

Add the garlic and onions to a large pot and sauté until softened.

Add the diced tomatoes, black beans, sweet potatoes, cumin, smoked paprika, chili powder, and salt and pepper.

Once the sweet potatoes are soft, simmer for 20 to 25 minutes.

Lemon Garlic Shrimp Stir-Fry

Ingredients:

1 pound shrimp (peeled and deveined)

2 cups broccoli florets

1 red bell pepper (sliced)

1 tablespoon olive oil

2 tablespoons soy sauce

2 tablespoons lemon juice

2 cloves garlic (minced)

1 teaspoon ginger (minced)

Brown rice (cooked, for serving)

Preparation:

Heat the olive oil in a wok or big skillet over medium-high heat.

Add shrimp, broccoli, and bell pepper. Stir-fry for 5-7 minutes until shrimp are cooked and vegetables are tender-crisp.

In a small bowl, mix soy sauce, lemon juice, minced garlic, and ginger. Pour over the shrimp and vegetables, stirring to coat.

Serve over cooked brown rice.

Greek Salad with Chickpeas

Ingredients:

2 cups cherry tomatoes (halved)

1 cucumber (diced)

1 can (15 oz) chickpeas (drained and rinsed)

1/2 cup Kalamata olives (pitted and sliced)

1/2 cup feta cheese (crumbled)

2 tablespoons olive oil

1 tablespoon red wine vinegar

1 teaspoon dried oregano

Salt and pepper to taste

Preparation:

Chickpeas, cucumber, feta, olives, and cherry tomatoes should all be combined in a big bowl.

Mix the olive oil, red wine vinegar, dried oregano, salt, and pepper in a small bowl.

Mix the salad and dressing until thoroughly mixed.

Pesto-crusted Zucchini Noodles with Cherry Tomatoes

Ingredients:

4 medium-sized zucchini (spiralized)

1 cup cherry tomatoes (halved)

1/2 cup fresh basil leaves

1/4 cup pine nuts

1/4 cup grated Parmesan cheese

2 cloves garlic (minced)

3 tablespoons olive oil

Salt and pepper to taste

Preparation:

In a blender or food processor, combine basil, pine nuts, Parmesan, garlic, and olive oil. Blend until smooth.

Toss spiralized zucchini and cherry tomatoes with the pesto.

Season with salt and pepper before serving.

Oven-Roasted Vegetables

Ingredients:
2 cups broccoli florets
2 cups cauliflower florets
2 carrots (cut into sticks)
1 red bell pepper (sliced)
1 tablespoon olive oil
1 teaspoon dried thyme
1 teaspoon dried rosemary
Salt and pepper to taste

Preparation:
Preheat the oven to 425°F (220°C).

In a large bowl, toss broccoli, cauliflower, carrots, and red bell pepper with olive oil, thyme, rosemary, salt, and pepper.

Spread vegetables on a baking sheet and roast for 20-25 minutes or until golden brown.

Stuffed Bell Peppers with Quinoa and Black Beans

Ingredients:
4 bell peppers (halved and seeds removed)
1 cup cooked quinoa
One can (15 oz) of rinsed and drained black beans
1 cup corn kernels (fresh or frozen)
1 cup salsa

1 teaspoon cumin

1/2 teaspoon chili powder

1/2 cup shredded cheddar cheese

Preparation:

Turn the oven on to 375°F, or 190°C.

Combine cooked quinoa, salsa, black beans, corn, cumin, and chili powder in a bowl.

Spoon mixture into bell pepper halves.

Add shredded cheddar cheese on top.

Bake peppers for 25 to 30 minutes, or until soft.

Mediterranean Chickpea Salad

Ingredients:

- One can (15 oz) of rinsed and drained chickpeas
- 1 cup cucumber (diced)
- 1 cup cherry tomatoes (halved)
- 1/2 cup red onion (finely chopped)
- 1/4 cup feta cheese (crumbled)
- 2 tablespoons olive oil
- 2 tablespoons lemon juice
- 1 teaspoon dried oregano
- Salt and pepper to taste

Preparation:

1. In a large bowl, combine chickpeas, cucumber, cherry tomatoes, red onion, and feta.

2. In a small bowl, whisk together olive oil, lemon juice, dried oregano, salt, and pepper.

3. Toss the salad with the dressing until well combined.

Lemon Garlic Roasted Chicken Thighs

Ingredients:
- 4 chicken thighs (bone-in, skin-on)
- 2 lemons (juiced)
- 4 cloves garlic (minced)
- 1 tablespoon olive oil
- 1 teaspoon dried thyme
- Salt and pepper to taste

Preparation:
1. Preheat the oven to 400°F (200°C).
2. In a small bowl, mix lemon juice, minced garlic, olive oil, dried thyme, salt, and pepper.
3. Place chicken thighs on a baking sheet and brush with the lemon-garlic mixture.
4. Roast for 30-35 minutes or until chicken is golden and cooked through.

Brown Rice and Black Bean Bowl

Ingredients:
- 2 cups cooked brown rice
- 1 can (15 oz) black beans (drained and rinsed)
- 1 cup corn kernels (fresh or frozen)
- 1 avocado (sliced)

- 1/4 cup cilantro (chopped)
- 1 lime (juiced)
- Salt and pepper to taste

Preparation:

1. In a bowl, combine cooked brown rice, black beans, corn, avocado, and cilantro.

2. Add a lime juice drizzle and season with pepper and salt.

3. Toss the ingredients together and serve.

Enjoy these delicious and nutritious DASH diet recipes!

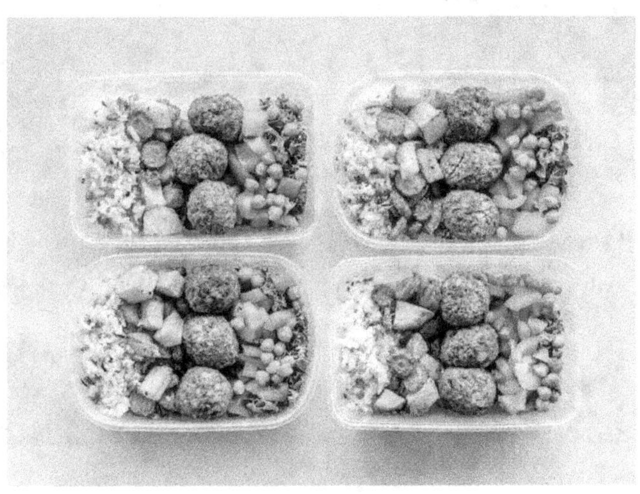

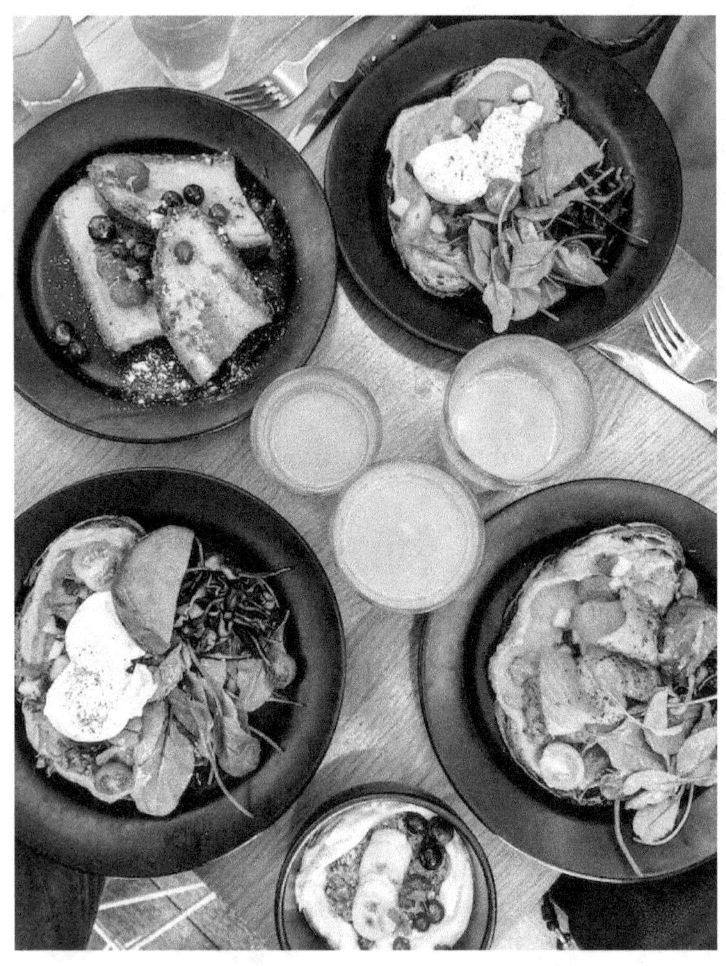

CHAPTER 4: VEGETARIAN WONDERS

Quinoa and Black Bean Salad:

Ingredients:
1 cup quinoa
1 can black beans, drained and rinsed
1 cup cherry tomatoes, halved
1 cucumber, diced
1/4 cup red onion, finely chopped
1/4 cup fresh cilantro, chopped
Juice of 2 limes
2 tablespoons olive oil
Salt and pepper to taste

Preparation:
As directed on the package, prepare the quinoa and allow it to cool.

Quinoa, black beans, cucumber, tomatoes, red onion, and cilantro should all be combined in a big bowl.

Mix the lime juice, olive oil, salt, and pepper in a small bowl.

After adding the dressing to the salad, gently toss to mix. Before serving, chill.

Vegetarian Chili:

Ingredients:
Two cans (15 oz each) of rinsed and drained black beans
One can (15 oz) of washed and drained kidney beans
1 can (28 oz) crushed tomatoes
1 cup corn kernels (fresh or frozen)
1 bell pepper, diced
1 onion, chopped
3 cloves garlic, minced
2 teaspoons chili powder
1 teaspoon cumin
Salt and pepper to taste

Preparation:
In a large pot, sauté onions, bell pepper, and garlic until softened.
Add beans, crushed tomatoes, corn, chili powder, cumin, salt, and pepper.
Bring to a boil, then reduce heat and simmer for 20-25 minutes.
Adjust seasoning as needed and serve hot.

Mediterranean Quinoa Salad:

Ingredients:
1 cup quinoa
1 cup cucumber, diced
1 cup cherry tomatoes, halved
1/2 cup Kalamata olives, sliced

1/2 cup feta cheese, crumbled

1/4 cup red onion, finely chopped

3 tablespoons olive oil

2 tablespoons red wine vinegar

1 teaspoon dried oregano

Salt and pepper to taste

Preparation:

As directed on the package, prepare the quinoa and allow it to cool.

Quinoa, cucumber, tomatoes, olives, feta, and red onion should all be combined in a big bowl.

Mix the olive oil, red wine vinegar, oregano, salt, and pepper in a small bowl.

After adding the dressing to the salad, gently toss to mix. Chill before serving.

Stuffed Bell Peppers:

Ingredients:

– 4 bell peppers, cut in half and seeded

– 1 cup cooked quinoa

_ One can (15 ounces) of rinsed and drained black beans

- One cup of frozen or fresh corn kernels

- 1 cup salsa

- 1 teaspoon cumin

- 1/2 teaspoon chili powder

- 1 cup shredded cheddar cheese (optional)

- Fresh cilantro for garnish

Preparation:

1. Preheat the oven to 375°F (190°C).

2. In a large bowl, combine cooked quinoa, black beans, corn, salsa, cumin, and chili powder.

3. Spoon the mixture into halved bell peppers and place them in a baking dish.

4. If desired, sprinkle shredded cheddar cheese on top.

5. Bake for 25-30 minutes or until peppers are tender.

6. Garnish with fresh cilantro before serving.

Spinach and Chickpea Stir-Fry:

Ingredients:

- 2 cups chickpeas, cooked or canned
- 4 cups fresh spinach
- 1 bell pepper, sliced
- 1 onion, thinly sliced
- 3 cloves garlic, minced
- 2 tablespoons olive oil
- 1 teaspoon cumin
- 1/2 teaspoon paprika
- Salt and pepper to taste

Preparation:

1. Heat the olive oil in a big skillet over medium heat.

2. Add garlic, bell pepper, and onion; sauté until softened.

3. Stir in chickpeas, spinach, cumin, paprika, salt, and pepper.

4. Cook until spinach wilts and chickpeas are heated through.

5. Adjust seasoning as needed and serve warm.

Eggplant and Tomato Bake:

Ingredients:
- 2 large eggplants, sliced
- 2 cups cherry tomatoes, halved
- 3 cloves garlic, minced
- 1/4 cup fresh basil, chopped
- 1/4 cup grated Parmesan cheese
- 2 tablespoons olive oil
- Salt and pepper to taste

Preparation:
1. Preheat the oven to 400°F (200°C).

2. Place the slices of eggplant on a baking pan and drizzle with olive oil.

3. In a bowl, combine cherry tomatoes, garlic, basil, Parmesan, salt, and pepper.

4. Spoon the tomato mixture over the eggplant slices.

5. Bake for 25-30 minutes or until the eggplant is tender.

6. Garnish with additional fresh basil before serving.

Enjoy these delicious and nutritious vegetarian DASH diet recipes!

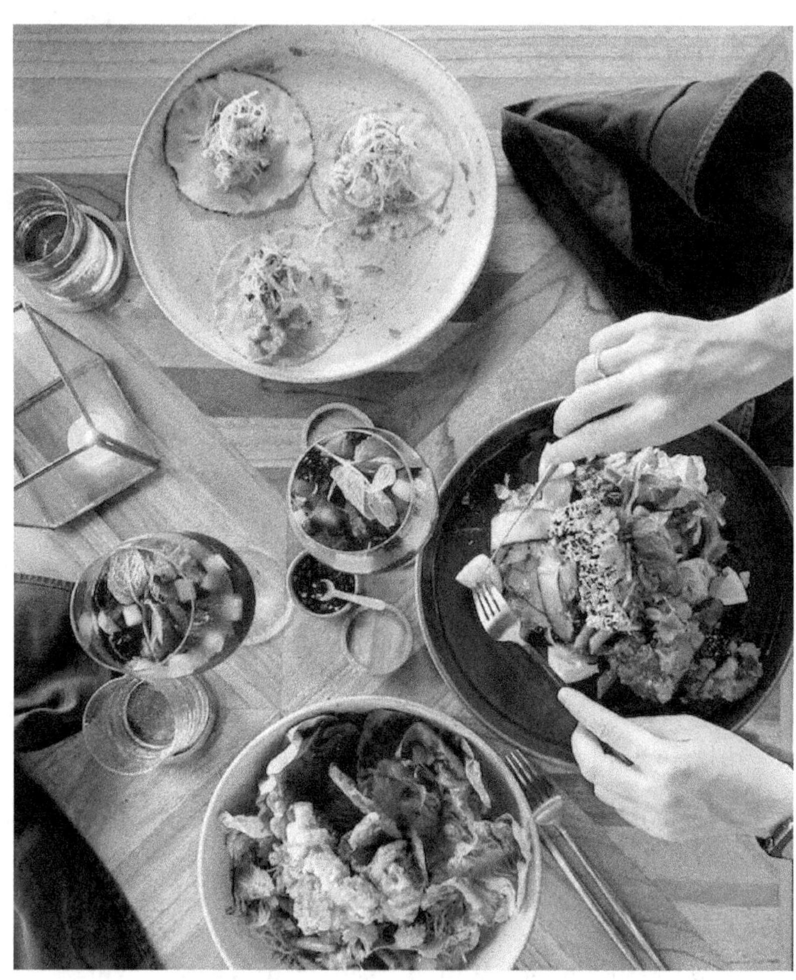

CHAPTER 5: SIDES AND SNACKS

Garlic Parmesan Roasted Brussels Sprouts

Ingredients:

1 pound Brussels sprouts, trimmed and halved

2 tablespoons olive oil

3 cloves garlic, minced

1/4 cup grated Parmesan cheese

Salt and pepper to taste

Instructions:

Set oven temperature to 400°F, or 200°C.

Brussels sprouts should be combined with olive oil, Parmesan cheese, minced garlic, salt, and pepper in a bowl.

Arrange the Brussels sprouts on a baking sheet so they are in a single layer.

Roast for 20 to 25 minutes, or until crispy and golden brown, in a preheated oven.

Enjoy it while it's hot!

Caprese Skewers

Ingredients:
Cherry tomatoes
Fresh mozzarella balls
Fresh basil leaves
Balsamic glaze
Toothpicks
Instructions:
Thread one cherry tomato, one mozzarella ball, and one basil leaf onto each toothpick.
Arrange the skewers on a serving platter.
Drizzle with balsamic glaze before serving.

Loaded Baked Potato Skins

Ingredients:
4 large russet potatoes
2 tablespoons olive oil
1 cup shredded cheddar cheese
1/2 cup sour cream
4 slices cooked bacon, crumbled
Chopped green onions for garnish
Instructions:
Preheat the oven to 400°F (200°C).

Bake potatoes until fork-tender. Cut in half and scoop out the flesh, leaving a thin layer.

Brush potato skins with olive oil and bake until crispy.

Fill each skin with cheese, bacon, and sour cream.

The cheese should be bubbling and melted after a few minutes under the broiler.

Garnish with chopped green onions and serve.

Spinach and Artichoke Dip

Ingredients:

1 (10 ounce) container of thawed and drained frozen chopped spinach

One can (14 oz) of drained and diced artichoke hearts

1 cup mayonnaise

1 cup sour cream

1 cup grated Parmesan cheese

1 cup shredded mozzarella cheese

2 cloves garlic, minced

Salt and pepper to taste

Instructions:

Preheat the oven to 375°F (190°C).

In a mixing bowl, combine spinach, artichoke hearts, mayonnaise, sour cream, Parmesan cheese, mozzarella cheese, garlic, salt, and pepper.

Transfer the mixture to a baking dish.

Bake for 25 to 30 minutes, or until bubbling and brown on top.

Serve with tortilla chips or sliced baguette.

Avocado and Black Bean Salsa

Ingredients:
2 avocados, diced
One can of (15 oz) black beans, drained and rinsed
1 cup corn kernels (fresh or frozen)
1 cup cherry tomatoes, halved
1/4 cup red onion, finely chopped
1/4 cup fresh cilantro, chopped
Juice of 2 limes
Salt and pepper to taste
Instructions:
In a large bowl, combine diced avocados, black beans, corn, cherry tomatoes, red onion, and cilantro.
Drizzle lime juice over the mixture and gently toss.
Season with salt and pepper to taste.
Let it cool for a minimum of half an hour before serving.

Buffalo Cauliflower Bites

Ingredients:
1 head cauliflower, cut into florets
1 cup flour
1 cup milk
1 cup buffalo sauce

2 tablespoons melted butter
1 teaspoon garlic powder
Ranch dressing for dipping

Instructions:

Preheat the oven to 450°F (230°C).

In a bowl, whisk together flour and milk to create a batter.

Dip each cauliflower floret into the batter, coating evenly, and place on a baking sheet.

Bake for 20-25 minutes or until crispy.

In a separate bowl, mix buffalo sauce, melted butter, and garlic powder.

Toss baked cauliflower in the buffalo sauce mixture until well coated.

Serve with ranch dressing for dipping

Sweet Potato Fries

Ingredients:

- Two large sweet potatoes, thinly sliced
- 2 tablespoons olive oil
- 1 teaspoon paprika
- 1 teaspoon garlic powder
- 1 teaspoon cumin
- Salt and pepper to taste

Instructions:

1. Preheat the oven to 425°F (220°C).

2. In a large bowl, toss sweet potato strips with olive oil, paprika, garlic powder, cumin, salt, and pepper until evenly coated.

3. Spread the sweet potato fries in a single layer on a baking sheet.

4. Bake for 20-25 minutes, flipping halfway through, or until fries are crispy and golden.

Bruschetta with Tomato and Basil

Ingredients:
- 4 large ripe tomatoes, diced
- 1/4 cup fresh basil, chopped
- 2 cloves garlic, minced
- 2 tablespoons balsamic vinegar
- 3 tablespoons olive oil
- Salt and pepper to taste
- Baguette slices, toasted

Instructions:
1. In a bowl, combine diced tomatoes, basil, minced garlic, balsamic vinegar, olive oil, salt, and pepper. Mix well.

2. Allow the mixture to marinate for at least 15 minutes.

3. Spoon the tomato and basil mixture onto toasted baguette slices.

4. Serve immediately.

Teriyaki Chicken Wing

Ingredients:
- 2 pounds chicken wings
- 1/2 cup soy sauce
- 1/4 cup honey
- 2 tablespoons rice vinegar
- 1 tablespoon sesame oil
- 2 cloves garlic, minced
- 1 teaspoon ginger, grated
- Sesame seeds and green onions for garnish

Instructions:

1. Preheat the oven to 400°F (200°C).

2. In a bowl, whisk together soy sauce, honey, rice vinegar, sesame oil, garlic, and ginger.

3. Place chicken wings in a large resealable plastic bag and pour half of the teriyaki sauce over them. Marinate for at least 30 minutes.

4. Bake the wings on a lined baking sheet for 45-50 minutes or until crispy.

5. Brush The remaining teriyaki sauce over the wings during the last 10 minutes of cooking.

6. Garnish with sesame seeds and chopped green onions before serving.

Cucumber Yogurt Dip (Tzatziki)

Ingredients:
- 1 cucumber, peeled, seeded, and finely diced

- 1 cup Greek yogurt

- 2 cloves garlic, minced

- 1 tablespoon fresh dill, chopped

- 1 tablespoon olive oil

- Salt and pepper to taste

Instructions:

1. In a bowl, combine diced cucumber, Greek yogurt, minced garlic, chopped dill, olive oil, salt, and pepper.

2. Thoroughly combine and chill for a minimum of 60 minutes prior to serving.

3. Serve the cucumber yogurt dip with pita bread or vegetable sticks.

Enjoy these delicious side dishes and snack recipes! Let me know if you have any more requests.

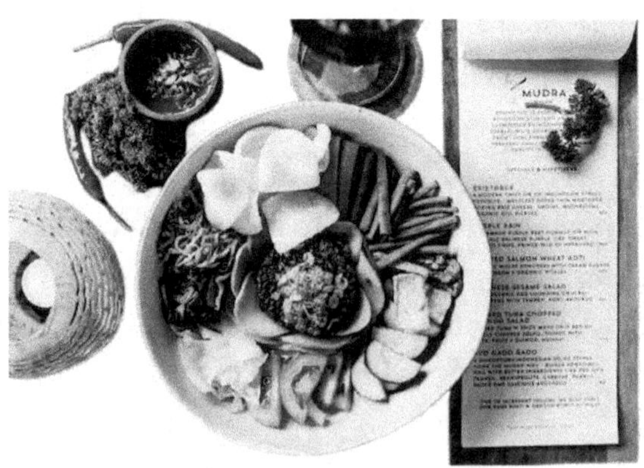

CHAPTER 6: DESSERTS

Chocolate Raspberry Truffle Tart:

Ingredients:
- 1 ½ cups chocolate cookie crumbs
- 6 tablespoons unsalted butter, melted
- 1 ½ cups dark chocolate chips
- 1 cup heavy cream
- 1 teaspoon vanilla extract
- 1 cup fresh raspberries

Instructions:
1. Preheat the oven to 350°F (175°C).
2. In a bowl, mix chocolate cookie crumbs and melted butter. To make the crust, press the mixture into a tart pan. After 8 minutes of baking, let it cool.
3. In a saucepan, heat the heavy cream until it simmers. Pour over the dark chocolate chips in a bowl. Stir until smooth. Add vanilla extract.
4. Pour the chocolate ganache into the cooled crust. Chill in the refrigerator for at least 2 hours.
5. Before serving, garnish with fresh raspberries.

Salted Caramel Pretzel Brownies:

Ingredients:
- One brownie mix box (comprising all ingredients specified on the package)

- 1 cup crushed pretzels
- 1 cup caramel sauce
- Sea salt for sprinkling

Instructions:

1. Prepare the brownie mix according to package instructions.

2. Fold in crushed pretzels into the brownie batter.

3. Pour half of the batter into a greased baking pan. Drizzle half of the caramel sauce.

4. Add the remaining batter and drizzle the rest of the caramel sauce. Use a toothpick to create a marbled effect.

5.Bake according per the brownie mix box's instructions. When finished, dust the top with sea salt. Before slicing into squares, allow it to cool.

Lemon Blueberry Cheesecake Parfait:

Ingredients:
- 1 ½ cups graham cracker crumbs
- ½ cup unsalted butter, melted
- 2 cups cream cheese, softened
- 1 cup powdered sugar
- 1 teaspoon vanilla extract
- Zest of 1 lemon
- 1 cup blueberries

Instructions:

1. Mix graham cracker crumbs with melted butter. Press into the bottom of serving glasses to create the crust.

2. In a bowl, beat cream cheese, powdered sugar, vanilla extract, and lemon zest until smooth.

3. Layer the cream cheese mixture over the crust in the glasses.

4. Top with fresh blueberries. Repeat the layers.

5. Refrigerate for at least 2 hours before serving.

Pistachio Chocolate Chip Ice Cream Sandwiches:

Ingredients:
- Pistachio ice cream
- Chocolate chip cookies (store-bought or homemade)

Instructions:

1. Allow the pistachio ice cream to soften slightly.

2. Spoon a generous scoop of ice cream onto the bottom side of one cookie.

3. Place another cookie on top, pressing down gently to create a sandwich.

4. Roll the edges of the ice cream sandwich in chocolate chips.

5. Freeze the sandwiches for at least 1 hour before serving.

Coconut Mango Rice Pudding:

Ingredients:
- 1 cup arborio rice
- 4 cups coconut milk
- 1 cup mango puree
- 1/2 cup sugar
- 1 teaspoon vanilla extract
- Shredded coconut for garnish

Instructions:

1. Put the rice and coconut milk in a saucepan. Once the rice is soft, cook it over medium heat.

2. Stir in mango puree, sugar, and vanilla extract. Cook for an additional 5 minutes.

3. Remove from heat and let it cool. Refrigerate for at least 2 hours.

4. Serve chilled, garnished with shredded coconut.

Berry-Lemon Mousse Cups:

Ingredients:
- 1 cup mixed berries (strawberries, blueberries, raspberries)
- 1 cup heavy cream
- 1/2 cup powdered sugar
- Zest and juice of 1 lemon
- 1 teaspoon gelatin powder (optional)

Instructions:

1. In a blender, puree half of the mixed berries. Strain to remove seeds, if desired.

2. If using gelatin, dissolve it in lemon juice and let it sit for a few minutes. Heat slightly to melt.

3. In a bowl, whip the heavy cream and powdered sugar until stiff peaks form.

4. Gently fold in the berry puree, lemon zest, and gelatin mixture.

5. Spoon the mousse into serving cups and refrigerate for at least 2 hours.

6. Top with the remaining mixed berries before serving.

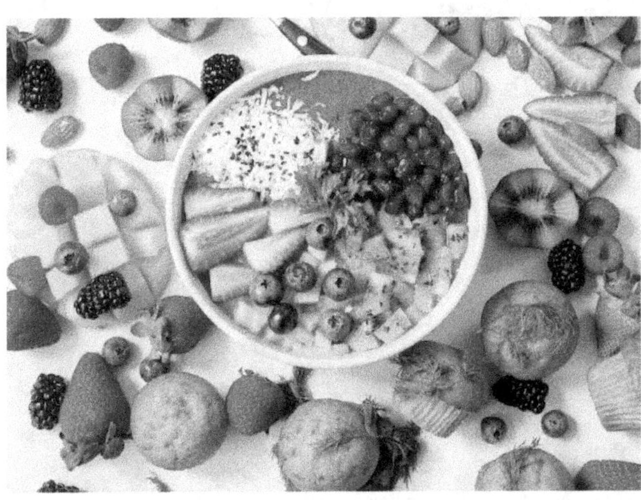

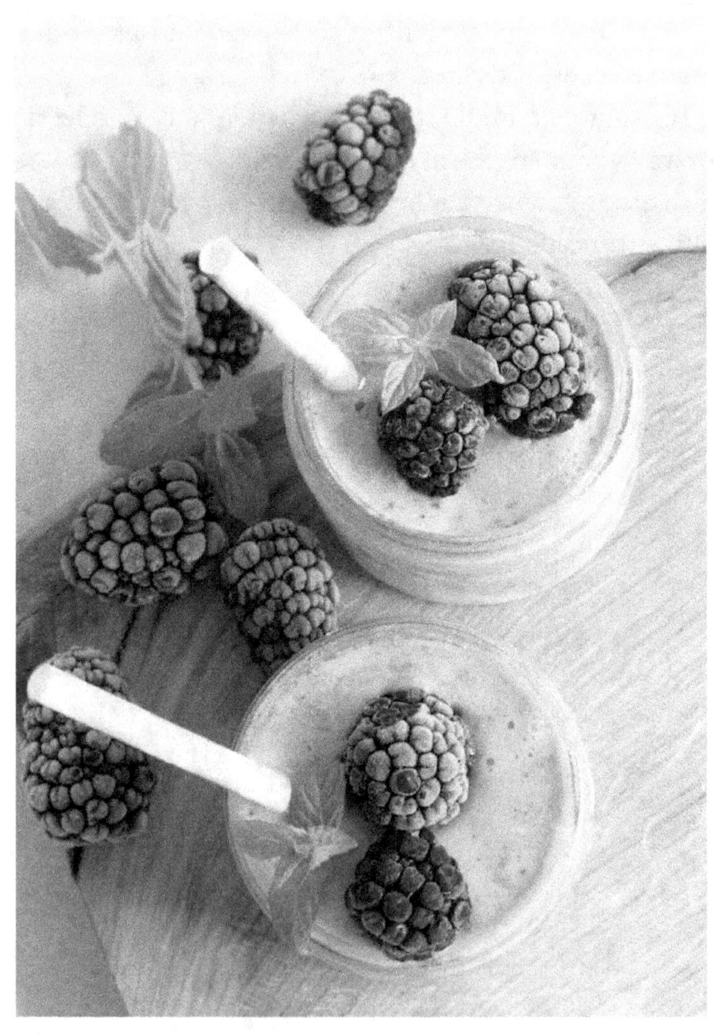

CHAPTER 7: BEVERAGES & SMOOTHIES

Classic Strawberry Banana Smoothie:

Ingredients:
- 1 cup frozen strawberries
- 1 ripe banana
- 1/2 cup yogurt
- 1/2 cup milk
- 1 tablespoon honey
- **Preparation:**
- Blend all ingredients until smooth. Serve chilled.

Green Detox Smoothie:

Ingredients:
- 1 cup spinach
- 1/2 cucumber, peeled and sliced
- 1/2 green apple, cored
- 1/2 lemon, juiced
- 1 cup coconut water
-**Preparation:**
- Combine all ingredients in a blender. Blend until well combined. Enjoy for a refreshing detox.

Tropical Paradise Smoothie:

- **Ingredients:**
  - 1/2 cup pineapple chunks
  - 1/2 cup mango chunks
  - 1/2 cup coconut milk
  - 1/2 cup orange juice
  - Ice cubes (optional)
- **Preparation:**
  - Mix every item until it's smooth. Transfer to a glass, and if preferred, top with ice cubes.
smooth. Pour into a glass and add ice cubes if desired.

Berry Blast Smoothie:

- **Ingredients:**
  - 1/2 cup blueberries
  - 1/2 cup raspberries
  - 1/2 cup strawberries
  - 1/2 cup Greek yogurt
  - 1 tablespoon chia seeds
- **Preparation:**
  - Blend berries, yogurt, and chia seeds until smooth. Garnish with extra berries or a sprinkle of chia seeds.

Mango Lassi:

- **Ingredients:**
  - 1 cup ripe mango, diced

- 1 cup yogurt
- 1/2 cup milk
- 1 tablespoon sugar (adjust to taste)
- A pinch of cardamom powder
- **Preparation:**
    - Blend all ingredients until smooth. Serve chilled, optionally garnished with a dash of cardamom on top.

Choco-Banana Protein Smoothie:

- **Ingredients:**
    - 1 ripe banana
    - 1 cup chocolate protein powder
    - 1 cup almond milk
    - 1 tablespoon peanut butter
    - Ice cubes (optional)
- **Preparation:**
    - Blend banana, protein powder, almond milk, and peanut butter until creamy. Add ice cubes for a colder treat.

Iced Matcha Latte:

- **Ingredients:**
    - 1 teaspoon matcha powder
    - 1 cup almond milk
    - 1 tablespoon honey
    - Ice cubes

- Preparation:

- Whisk matcha powder with a little hot water until smooth. Add honey and almond milk. Pour over ice.

Pineapple Ginger Mint Refresher:

-Ingredients:

- 1 cup pineapple chunks
- 1 teaspoon grated ginger
- A handful of fresh mint leaves
- 1 tablespoon honey
- 1 cup coconut water

- Preparation:

- Blend pineapple, ginger, mint, honey, and coconut water until well combined. Strain if desired.

Cucumber Mint Cooler:

- Ingredients:

- 1/2 cucumber, sliced
- A handful of fresh mint leaves
- 1 tablespoon lemon juice
- 1 tablespoon agave syrup
- 1 cup sparkling water

- Preparation:

- Muddle cucumber, mint, lemon juice, and agave syrup. Add ice and top with sparkling water. Stir gently.

Avocado Banana Smoothie:

- **Ingredients:**
  - 1 ripe avocado
  - 1 ripe banana
  - 1/2 cup spinach
  - 1 cup almond milk
  - 1 tablespoon chia seeds
- **Preparation:**
  - Blend avocado, banana, spinach, almond milk, and chia seeds until creamy. Pour into a glass and enjoy.

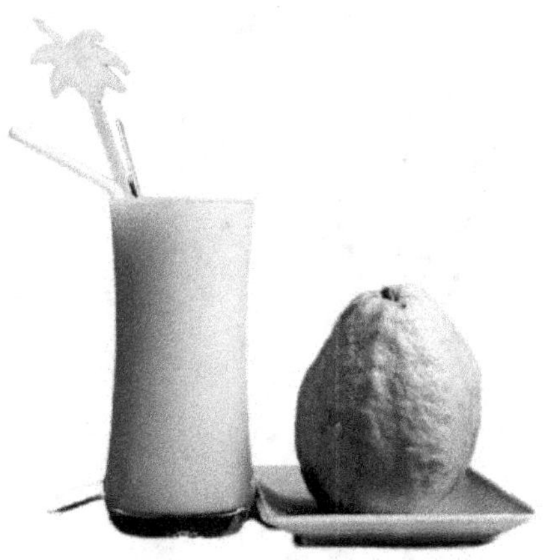

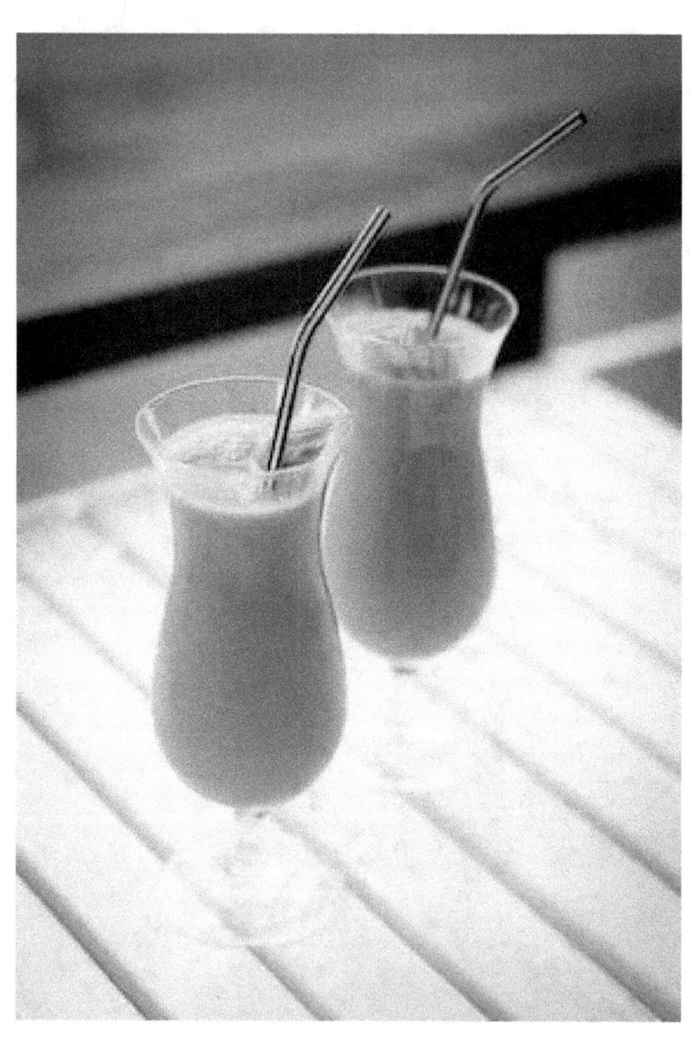

CHAPTER 8: MEAL PLANNING AND TIPS

Weekly Meal Planner

A dietary regimen called the DASH (Dietary Approaches to Stop Hypertension) diet is intended to help control and prevent hypertension, or high blood pressure. It emphasizes the consumption of nutrient-rich foods that are low in sodium. Here's a sample weekly meal planner for the DASH diet:

Day 1:

- **Breakfast:**
  - Berries with Greek yogurt with a honey drizzle
  - Whole-grain toast with avocado
- **Lunch:**
  - Grilled chicken salad with mixed vegetables, olive oil, and lemon dressing
  - Quinoa on the side
- **Snack:**
  - Apple slices with a tablespoon of almond butter
- **Dinner:**
  - Baked salmon with a lemon squeeze
  - Steamed broccoli and carrots
  - Brown rice

Day 2:

- **Breakfast:**
  - Banana slices mixed with oatmeal and chia seeds
  - Low-fat milk or plant-based milk
- **Lunch**:
  - Lentil soup
  - Whole-grain pita bread
  - Cherry tomatoes with a mixed green salad dressed with a balsamic vinaigrette
- **Snack**:
  - Carrot and cucumber sticks with hummus
- **Dinner**:
  - Turkey meatballs with tomato sauce
  - Whole-grain pasta
  - Roasted Brussels sprouts

Day 3:

- **Breakfast:**
  - Smoothie with spinach, berries, banana, and low-fat yogurt
  - Whole-grain toast with peanut butter
- **Lunch:**
  - Quinoa and black bean bowl with salsa
  - Mixed greens salad with avocado
- **Snack:**
  - Greek yogurt with a handful of nuts
- **Dinner:**

- Grilled shrimp with lemon and herbs
- Sweet potato wedges
- Asparagus spears

Day 4:

- **Breakfast:**
  - Scrambled eggs with spinach and feta cheese
  - Whole-grain English muffin
- **Lunch:**
  - Tuna salad with mixed greens
  - Brown rice cakes
- **Snack:**
  - Fresh fruit salad
- **Dinner:**
  - Baked chicken breast with rosemary and garlic
  - Quinoa pilaf
  - Steamed green beans

Day 5:

- **Breakfast:**
  - Whole-grain pancakes with fresh berries
  - Low-fat yogurt
- **Lunch:**
  - Chickpea and vegetable stir-fry
  - Brown rice
- **Snack:**

  - Cottage cheese with pineapple chunks
- **Dinner:**
  - Grilled cod with lemon and dill
  - Couscous
  - Roasted mixed vegetables

Day 6:

- **Breakfast:**
  - Whole-grain waffles topped with fresh berries
  - Low-fat Greek yogurt
- **Lunch:**
  - Quinoa salad with diced tomatoes, cucumbers, feta cheese, and olives
  - Grilled chicken breast slices
- **Snack:**
  - Pear slices with a few walnuts
- **Dinner:**
  - Baked tilapia with a squeeze of lime
  - Wild rice
  - Steamed asparagus

Day 7:

- **Breakfast:**
  - Vegetable omelet with mushrooms, bell peppers, and spinach
  - Whole-grain toast with avocado

- Lunch:
 - Lentil and vegetable wrap with whole-grain tortilla
 - Mixed green salad with a light vinaigrette
- Snack:
 - A small handful of cherry tomatoes with mozzarella cheese
- Dinner:
 - Grilled vegetable and quinoa-stuffed bell peppers
 - Roasted sweet potato wedges
 - Steamed broccoli

Remember to adapt these meals to your personal preferences and dietary requirements. It's also important to stay consistent with the DASH diet principles, including limiting sodium intake, incorporating lean protein sources, and emphasizing fruits, vegetables, whole grains, and low-fat dairy. Additionally, consider spreading your meals throughout the day to maintain energy levels and prevent excessive hunger.

SHOPPING LIST ESSENTIALS

The DASH (Dietary Approaches to Stop Hypertension) diet is designed to help prevent and manage high blood pressure. It emphasizes the consumption of nutrient-rich foods that are low in sodium. Here's a shopping list of essentials for the DASH diet:

Fruits:
- Apples
- Berries (strawberries, blueberries, raspberries)
- Bananas
- Oranges
- Grapefruit
- Peaches
- Pears

Vegetables:
- Leafy greens (spinach, kale, collard greens)
- Broccoli
- Carrots
- Bell peppers
- Tomatoes
- Sweet potatoes
- Zucchini

Whole Grains:
- Brown rice
- Quinoa
- Oats
- Whole wheat bread

  - Whole wheat pasta
  - Barley

Lean Proteins:
  - Skinless poultry (chicken, turkey)
  - Fish (salmon, trout, tuna)
  - Lean cuts of beef or pork
  - Tofu
  - Legumes (beans, lentils)

Dairy or Dairy Alternatives:
  - Low-fat or fat-free milk
  - Greek yogurt
  - Cheese (in moderation)
  - Almond or soy milk (unsweetened)

Nuts and Seeds:
  - Almonds
  - Walnuts
  - Chia seeds
  - Flaxseeds

Healthy Fats:
  - Olive oil
  - Avocados
  - Canola oil

Snacks:
  - Hummus
  - Air-popped popcorn (without excessive butter or salt)
  - Fresh fruit

Herbs and Spices:
- Garlic
- Basil
- Oregano
- Rosemary
- Cinnamon
- Dill
- Cumin

Beverages:
- Water
- Herbal tea (unsweetened)
- Coffee (in moderation)
- Limited sodium vegetable juice

Limit or Avoid:
- High-sodium processed foods
- Sugary beverages
- Saturated and trans fats
- Excessive red meat

Remember to always consult with a healthcare professional or a registered dietitian before making significant changes to your diet, especially if you have specific health concerns or conditions.

DASH Diet Cooking Techniques

Grilling and Broiling:

- Use these methods to cook lean proteins such as skinless poultry, fish, and lean cuts of meat.

- Avoid adding excessive amounts of salt or high-sodium marinades. Instead, use herbs, spices, and citrus for flavor.

Steaming:

- Steaming is a healthy cooking method that helps preserve the nutrients in vegetables, fish, and other foods.

- Season with herbs, lemon, or vinegar instead of salt.

Baking and Roasting:

- Choose baking or roasting for poultry, fish, and vegetables.

- Use herbs, garlic, onions, and other flavorful ingredients to enhance taste without relying on salt.

Sautéing:

- Use heart-healthy oils like olive oil for sautéing.

- Add garlic, onions, and a variety of herbs for flavor instead of excessive salt.

Stir-Frying:

- Stir-frying is a quick and efficient way to cook vegetables and lean proteins.

- Use minimal oil and opt for a variety of colorful vegetables to maximize nutrients.

Herb and Spice Blends:

- Create your own herb and spice blends to season foods without relying on salt.

- Experiment with combinations like garlic, thyme, rosemary, basil, and more to add depth of flavor.

Fresh Citrus Juices:

- Use fresh lemon or lime juice to add a burst of flavor to salads, vegetables, and grilled proteins.

- Citrus can enhance taste without the need for additional salt.

Low-Sodium Broths and Stocks:

- Choose low-sodium or sodium-free broths and stocks for soups, stews, and sauces.

- Add a variety of vegetables, beans, and lean proteins for a nutrient-rich meal.

Limiting Processed Foods:

- Minimize the use of processed and pre-packaged foods, as they often contain high levels of sodium.

- Opt for fresh, whole ingredients whenever possible.

Experiment with Fresh Herbs:

- Fresh herbs like parsley, cilantro, basil, and dill can add vibrancy and flavor to dishes without the need for excess salt.

Kitchen Tools for DASH Diet Cooking

Food Scale:

- Useful for measuring portion sizes and ensuring accurate ingredient amounts.

Measuring Cups and Spoons:

- For precise measurement of ingredients, especially when following specific recipes.

Steamer Basket:

- Ideal for cooking vegetables without losing their nutritional value. Steaming helps retain nutrients better than boiling.

Non-Stick Cookware:

- Reduces the need for excessive cooking oils or fats.

Food Processor or Blender:

- Useful for preparing homemade sauces, dips, and smoothies using fresh and healthy ingredients.

Herb and Spice Grinder:

- Enhances flavor without the need for excessive salt. Freshly ground herbs and spices can add depth to your dishes.

Citrus Juicer:

- Enables you to add fresh citrus juice to recipes for flavor without relying on salt.

Grill Pan:

- Provides a way to cook lean proteins like chicken or fish without adding extra fat.

Olive Oil Mister:

- Allows you to control the amount of oil you use when cooking. Olive oil is a heart-healthy choice in moderation.

Salad Spinner:

- Makes it easy to wash and spin-dry fresh vegetables for salads without adding excess moisture.

Non-Stick Baking Sheets:

- Useful for roasting vegetables or baking whole grains without the need for excessive oils.

Zester/Grater:

- Helps you incorporate the flavor of citrus peels or ginger into your dishes, adding taste without salt.

Sharp Chef's Knife:

- A good-quality knife makes it easier to cut and prepare fresh fruits and vegetables.

Vegetable Spiralizer:

- Allows you to create vegetable "noodles" from zucchini or other veggies, providing a healthy alternative to traditional pasta.

Food Storage Containers:

- Essential for storing prepped ingredients and leftovers, promoting portion control.

SPECIAL OCCASION MENUS

DASH Diet-Friendly Holiday Feast

Creating a DASH diet-friendly holiday feast involves incorporating the principles of the DASH diet while still enjoying a delicious and festive meal. Here's a suggested menu for a DASH diet-friendly holiday feast:

Appetizers:

1. Vegetable Platter with Hummus:

- Assorted colorful veggies like bell peppers, cucumbers, and cherry tomatoes with a side of homemade hummus.

2. Caprese Skewers:

- Balsamic-glazed kebabs topped with cherry tomatoes, fresh mozzarella, and basil.

Main Course:

Herb-Roasted Turkey:

- Roast turkey seasoned with herbs like rosemary, thyme, and sage. Avoid excessive salt and use herbs for flavor.

4. Baked Salmon:

- A flavorful salmon dish with a lemon and dill marinade.

5. Quinoa and Vegetable Stuffed Acorn Squash:

- Acorn squash halves filled with a stuffing made from quinoa, sautéed vegetables, and herbs.

Side Dishes:

6. Garlic Mashed Cauliflower:

- A low-carb alternative to mashed potatoes, using cauliflower mashed with garlic and a touch of olive oil.

7. Roasted Brussels Sprouts:

- Brussels sprouts roasted with a drizzle of olive oil, garlic, and a sprinkle of parmesan.

8. Cranberry Orange Quinoa Salad:

- A refreshing salad with quinoa, cranberries, orange segments, and a light vinaigrette.

9. Sweet Potato Casserole:

- Mashed sweet potatoes with a topping made from chopped nuts, a hint of cinnamon, and a touch of maple syrup.

Desserts:

10. Fresh Fruit Salad:

- A medley of seasonal fresh fruits for a light and naturally sweet dessert.

11. Greek Yogurt Parfait:

- Layered Greek yogurt with berries and a sprinkle of nuts for added texture.

12. Pumpkin Chia Seed Pudding:

- A healthy pumpkin-flavored chia seed pudding sweetened with a touch of maple syrup.

Beverages:

13. Infused Water or Herbal Tea:

   - Offer infused water with citrus slices or herbal tea as a refreshing and hydrating option.

Tips for DASH Diet-Friendly Cooking:

- Use herbs and spices to flavor dishes instead of relying on excessive salt.

- Choose lean proteins like turkey, salmon, and legumes.

- Incorporate a variety of colorful vegetables for a range of nutrients.

- Opt for whole grains like quinoa instead of refined grains.

- Limit added sugars, and choose natural sweeteners if needed.

By focusing on whole, nutrient-dense foods and mindful preparation, you can create a festive holiday feast that aligns with the DASH diet principles while still being enjoyable for everyone at the table.

Celebratory Dinner Party Menu

A celebratory dinner party menu can be a delightful combination of flavors and textures. Here's a suggestion for a three-course menu:

Appetizers:

1. Stuffed Mushrooms:
  - Mushrooms packed with breadcrumbs, cream cheese, garlic, and spices.
  - Baked until golden and delicious.

2. Shrimp Cocktail:
  - Chilled shrimp served with a tangy cocktail sauce.
  - Garnish with lemon wedges and fresh parsley.

Main Course:

3. Filet Mignon with Red Wine Reduction:
  - Tender filet mignon steaks cooked to perfection.
  - Drizzled with a rich red wine reduction sauce.
  - Served with roasted vegetables or asparagus.

4. Lemon Herb Roasted Chicken:
  - Chicken marinated in a blend of herbs and lemon
- Roasted to a golden brown color and then presented with a thin pan sauce.

5. Truffle Mashed Potatoes:
  - Creamy mashed potatoes infused with truffle oil for an elegant touch.

6. Grilled Vegetable Medley:
  - A colorful mix of seasonal vegetables grilled to perfection.

Dessert:

7. Chocolate Fondue:

- A decadent chocolate fondue served with a variety of dippable items like strawberries, marshmallows, and pretzels.

8. Classic Vanilla Crème Brûlée:

- Creamy vanilla custard with a crisp caramelized sugar crust.

Beverages:

9. Sparkling Cranberry Punch:

- A refreshing non-alcoholic punch made with sparkling water, cranberry juice, and a hint of citrus.

10. Wine Pairing:

- Offer a selection of red and white wines to complement the main course.

Coffee and Digestifs:

11. Gourmet Coffee Bar:

- Provide a selection of gourmet coffees and teas.

12. Digestifs:

- Offer a variety of after-dinner drinks, such as port wine, brandy, or liqueurs.

Adjust portion sizes based on the number of guests, and don't forget to enjoy the celebration!

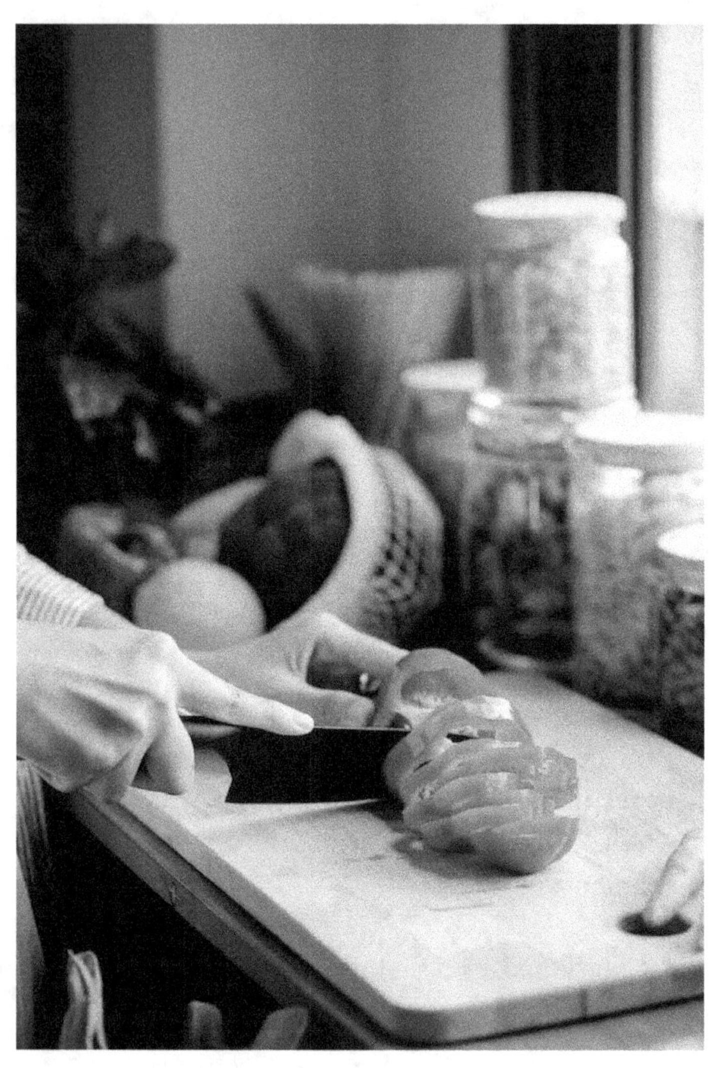

RESOURCES AND REFERENCES

Recommended Reading

The Dietary Approaches to Stop Hypertension (DASH) diet is a dietary plan designed to help prevent and manage hypertension (high blood pressure). Here are some recommended readings to learn more about the DASH diet:

1. "The DASH Diet Action Plan" by Marla Heller, MS, RD:** This book provides a comprehensive guide to the DASH diet, offering practical tips, recipes, and a 28-day meal plan to help you implement the dietary changes.

2. "The DASH Diet Weight Loss Solution" by Marla Heller, MS, RD: Another book by Marla Heller, this one focuses on combining the principles of the DASH diet with weight loss strategies. It includes meal plans, recipes, and exercise tips.

3. "DASH Diet for Beginners" by John Chatham: This beginner-friendly guide introduces the basics of the DASH diet, including its principles and benefits. It also includes simple recipes to get you started.

4. "The Complete DASH Diet for Beginners" by Jennifer Koslo, PhD, RD, CSSD: This book provides a thorough introduction to the DASH diet, including its health benefits and practical tips for implementation. It also features a 14-day meal plan.

5. "DASH Diet Cookbook" by Serena Ball, MS, RD, and Deanna Segrave-Daly, RD: A cookbook tailored to the DASH diet, This source provides a range of appetizing and nourishing meals that follow the diet's guidelines.

6. "The DASH Diet Mediterranean Solution" by Marla Heller, MS, RD: This book combines the DASH diet with the Mediterranean diet, offering a flexible and flavorful approach to heart-healthy eating.

Remember to consult with a healthcare professional or a registered dietitian before making significant changes to your diet, especially if you have any pre-existing health conditions.

Online Cooking Resources

If you're looking for online resources to find DASH diet-friendly recipes and cooking inspiration, there are several websites and platforms that offer a variety of recipes and meal ideas. Here are some online resources for DASH diet cooking:

1. American Heart Association (AHA) - DASH Recipes:
- [AHA DASH Recipes](https://recipes.heart.org/en/recipes): The American Heart Association provides a collection of DASH diet recipes on its website. You can find breakfast, lunch, dinner, and snack ideas that adhere to DASH diet principles.

2. National Heart, Lung, and Blood Institute (NHLBI) - Your Guide to Lowering Your Blood Pressure with DASH:
- [NHLBI DASH Recipes](https://www.nhlbi.nih.gov/health-topics/dash-eating-plan#recipes): The NHLBI offers a variety of DASH diet recipes on its website. You can explore different categories such as main dishes, salads, and desserts.

3. Mayo Clinic - DASH Diet Recipes:

- [Mayo Clinic DASH Recipes](https://www.mayoclinic.org/healthy-lifestyle/nutrition-and-healthy-eating/in-depth/dash-diet/art-20047110): Mayo Clinic provides a selection of DASH diet recipes along with nutritional information and cooking tips.

4. EatingWell - DASH Diet Recipes:

- [EatingWell DASH Recipes](https://www.eatingwell.com/category/4303/dash-diet/): EatingWell offers a dedicated section for DASH diet recipes. You can find a variety of dishes, each with clear instructions and nutritional details.

5. Allrecipes - DASH Diet Recipes:

- [Allrecipes DASH Recipes](https://www.allrecipes.com/recipes/15957/healthy-recipes/dash/): Allrecipes has a collection of DASH diet recipes contributed by users. You can explore and try out recipes rated and reviewed by others.

6. Cooking Light - DASH Diet Recipes:

- [Cooking Light DASH Recipes](https://www.cookinglight.com/eating-smart/nutrition-101/dash-diet-recipes): Cooking Light provides a variety of DASH diet recipes, often focusing on lighter and healthier versions of classic dishes.

Consultation with Nutritionists and Dietitians

If you're considering a consultation with a nutritionist or dietitian, it's a great step toward obtaining personalized advice and guidance for your dietary needs and health goals. Here are some steps to help you find and schedule a consultation:

Ask for Recommendations:

- Seek recommendations from your primary care physician, friends, family, or colleagues. They may know of reputable nutritionists or dietitians in your area.

Check Credentials:

- Look for professionals who are registered dietitians (RD) or nutritionists with relevant certifications. Credentials ensure that the individual has undergone the necessary education and training.

Use Online Directories:

- Websites like the Academy of Nutrition and Dietetics (eatright.org) provide directories where you can search for registered dietitians in your location.

Check Reviews:

- Read reviews and testimonials from previous clients if available. This can give you an idea of the professional's approach and effectiveness.

Contact Health Insurance:

- If you have health insurance, check if nutrition consultations are covered. Some insurance plans may cover a certain number of sessions with a registered dietitian.

Schedule a Consultation:

- Once you've identified potential professionals, contact them to inquire about their availability and schedule a consultation. Some dietitians may offer virtual consultations as well.

Prepare for the Consultation:

- Before the consultation, make a list of your health goals, dietary preferences, any medical conditions, and questions you may have. This information will help the nutritionist or dietitian provide tailored advice.

During the Consultation:

- Be open and honest about your lifestyle, eating habits, and any challenges you face. The more information you provide, the better the professional can tailor their recommendations to your needs.

Follow-Up and Adjustments:

- After the initial consultation, the nutritionist or dietitian may provide a plan or recommendations. Follow up as recommended, and discuss any challenges or successes. They can make adjustments to your plan based on your progress.

Remember that the information you share during a consultation is confidential, and the professional is there to help you make positive and sustainable changes to your diet and lifestyle. Regular follow-up sessions may be recommended to track progress and make any necessary adjustments to your plan.

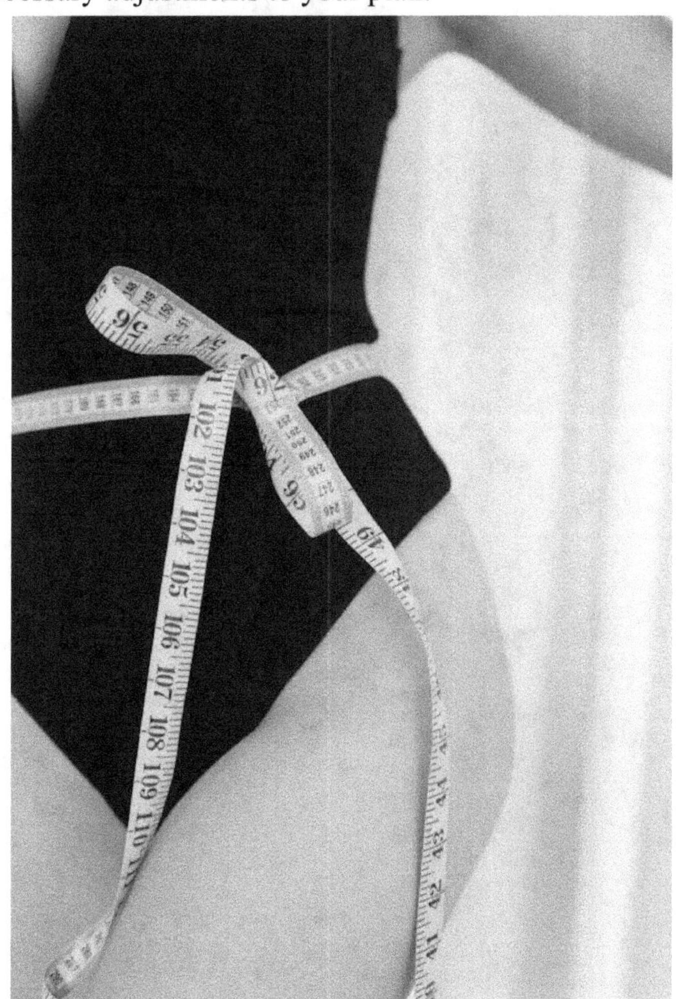

HAPPY

NEW

YEAR!!